Chair yoga for men over 50

Rediscover Vitality, Strength, and Inner Balance with Gentle Chair Yoga Practices Tailored for Men in their Prime Years (50,60, 70)

Maxwell Strong

Scan the code to download bonus

Table of Contents

INTRODUCTION

Ditch the aches, discover the gains: Chair Yoga for Men Over 50 - Your Gateway to Strength, Balance, and Zen.

Turning 50? It's not just a milestone, it's a rebirth. Forget slowing down, embrace rediscovering your peak, with a little help from your trusty chair. This book is your go-to guide to chair yoga, the practice designed specifically for men like you.

No matter your fitness level, experience, or aches and pains, chair yoga is about feeling good, moving freely, and laughing at limitations. This book doesn't just promise strength and flexibility, it delivers science-backed secrets on how chair yoga transforms your body and mind.

Remember Mark? The guy from work who always seemed grumpy, riddled with back pain, and perpetually glued to his office chair? Yeah, him. Turns out, Mark wasn't grumpy, just stiff and frustrated. At 52, his body was protesting – aches in his back, knees clicking like rusty hinges, and the thought of joining a "regular" yoga class made him sweat more than the poses themselves.

Then he heard about chair yoga. He scoffed at first, but desperation and a nagging wife led him to give it a try. Sitting down for yoga? Ridiculous, right? **Wrong.**

From the first gentle stretch, Mark felt a release. His tight muscles loosened, his breath deepened, and a surprising giggle escaped his lips. Turns out, moving even seated felt good! Over the next few weeks, as he followed the tailored routines in this book, something amazing happened. Mark wasn't just more flexible, he felt stronger, calmer, and even dared we say, happier. His backache vanished, his energy soared, and he found himself laughing more – not just at himself in the mirror, but at life in general.

Chair yoga wasn't just exercise; it was a revelation. It was a community of men, just like him, rediscovering their bodies and their zest for life. It was stress relief, pain management, and a surprising dose of fun, all from the comfort of… **you guessed it right, a chair!**

Ready to rewrite your own story? Grab your chair, open this book, and say goodbye to limitations. Chair yoga awaits!

Yoga is often associated with flexibility, meditation, and spirituality, but its benefits extend far beyond these surface-level perceptions. For men over 50, incorporating yoga into their lifestyle can be a game-changer, offering a multitude of physical, mental, and emotional advantages. Here's a closer look at the remarkable benefits of yoga for men in their prime years:

- **Improved Flexibility and Mobility:** As men age, flexibility tends to decline, leading to stiffness and reduced range of motion. Yoga helps counteract this by gently stretching and lengthening muscles, ligaments, and tendons, improving overall flexibility and mobility. This enhanced flexibility not only aids in daily activities but also reduces the risk of injuries and promotes better posture.

- **Enhanced Strength and Muscle Tone:** Contrary to popular belief, yoga is not just about stretching—it also builds strength. Many yoga poses require participants to engage and stabilize various muscle groups, leading to improved muscle tone and overall strength. For men over 50, maintaining muscle mass is crucial for preventing age-related muscle loss and preserving functional independence.

- **Better Balance and Stability:** Balance and stability become increasingly important as we age, helping to prevent falls and maintain independence. Yoga poses often involve shifting weight and practicing proprioception, which enhances balance and stability. This is especially beneficial for older adults who may be at higher risk of falls due to factors like decreased muscle strength and impaired balance.

- **Pain Relief and Management:** Chronic pain is a common issue among older adults, affecting quality of life and daily functioning. Yoga has been shown to alleviate various types of pain, including back pain, arthritis, and joint discomfort. Through gentle stretching, strengthening, and mindful movement, yoga helps reduce pain, improve flexibility, and enhance overall physical comfort.

- **Stress Reduction and Relaxation:** The practice of yoga emphasizes deep breathing, mindfulness, and relaxation techniques, which can significantly reduce stress levels and promote a sense of calmness and inner peace. For men navigating the challenges of career, family, and aging, yoga provides a sanctuary for stress relief, allowing them to unwind, recharge, and cultivate mental resilience.

- **Mental Clarity and Cognitive Function:** Yoga isn't just beneficial for the body—it also nourishes the mind. Regular yoga practice has been linked to improved cognitive function, memory, and mental clarity. By quieting the mind, reducing stress, and promoting mindfulness, yoga enhances focus, concentration, and cognitive performance, helping men over 50 stay sharp and mentally agile.

- **Emotional Wellbeing and Resilience:** Yoga offers a holistic approach to emotional health, supporting men in navigating life's ups and downs with greater resilience and equanimity. Through introspection, self-awareness, and acceptance, yoga fosters emotional balance, self-confidence, and a deeper connection to oneself and others. This emotional resilience becomes especially valuable as men navigate the transitions and challenges of midlife and beyond.

Why Chair Yoga?

Chair yoga is a gentle form of yoga practice that adapts traditional yoga poses and techniques to be performed while seated on a chair or using a chair for support. It offers a modified approach to yoga, making it accessible to individuals of all ages, abilities, and fitness levels.

Chair yoga has gained popularity in recent years as a gentle yet effective form of yoga practice that offers numerous benefits for people of all ages and abilities. Whether you're a seasoned yogi looking for a low-impact option or a beginner seeking a accessible way to incorporate yoga into your routine, chair yoga provides a wealth of advantages that make it a compelling choice. Let's delve into some of the reasons why you should consider embracing chair yoga.

One of the most significant advantages of chair yoga is its accessibility. Unlike traditional yoga, which often involves getting down on the floor and maneuvering into various poses, chair yoga can be practiced entirely from a seated position. This makes it an ideal option for individuals with mobility issues, chronic pain, or other physical limitations, allowing them to experience the benefits of yoga without discomfort or difficulty.

Chair yoga provides a stable and supportive environment for practicing yoga poses, reducing the risk of injury and strain. The chair serves as a prop, offering stability and balance during poses, making it easier to maintain proper alignment and posture. This added support is particularly beneficial for older adults or those recovering from injury, providing a safe and comfortable way to engage in yoga practice.

Despite being seated, chair yoga offers a surprising range of motion and flexibility benefits. The gentle stretching and movement sequences target key muscle groups, joints, and connective tissues, helping to improve flexibility, range of motion, and joint mobility. Over time, regular practice can lead to increased suppleness and ease of movement, enhancing overall physical comfort and function.

While chair yoga may seem less physically demanding than traditional yoga, it still offers opportunities for strength building and muscle engagement. Many chair yoga poses require participants to engage their core, stabilize their spine, and activate various muscle groups, leading to improved strength and muscle tone. This is particularly beneficial for older adults who may be at risk of age-related muscle loss and weakness.

Like all forms of yoga, chair yoga emphasizes deep breathing, mindfulness, and relaxation techniques, promoting a sense of calmness and relaxation. By focusing on the breath and tuning into the present moment, chair yoga helps reduce stress, anxiety, and tension, fostering a greater sense of inner peace and emotional wellbeing. This makes it an excellent option for anyone seeking stress relief or relaxation in their daily life.

Despite its seated nature, chair yoga encourages a deep connection between the mind and body, fostering greater self-awareness and mindfulness. Through focused attention and intentional movement, practitioners learn to listen to their bodies, honor their limitations, and cultivate a sense of acceptance and compassion towards themselves. This mind-body connection can have profound effects on overall wellbeing, promoting greater resilience, self-confidence, and inner harmony.

Chair yoga is incredibly versatile and can be adapted to suit a wide range of needs, preferences, and fitness levels. Whether you're recovering from injury, managing a chronic condition, or simply looking for a gentle way to stay active, chair yoga can be customized to meet your individual needs and goals. From gentle stretching to more dynamic movement sequences, there's something for everyone in chair yoga.

Scan Code to download free Bonus

Chapter 1

History and Origins of Chair Yoga

Chair yoga traces its roots back to the ancient practice of yoga, which originated in India over 5,000 years ago. While traditional yoga typically involves a combination of physical postures (asanas), breathing exercises (pranayama), and meditation (dhyana), chair yoga emerged as a modified form of yoga to accommodate individuals with mobility issues, injuries, or other limitations.

The precise origins of chair yoga are difficult to pinpoint, but it gained traction in the West during the late 20th century as yoga gained popularity as a holistic wellness practice. In the United States, yoga teachers and healthcare professionals began to recognize the need for modifications to make yoga accessible to diverse populations, leading to the development of chair yoga as a specialized practice.

Over the years, chair yoga has evolved and diversified, with various teachers and practitioners contributing their expertise and creativity to the field. Today, chair yoga is widely practiced in community centers, senior centers, hospitals, rehabilitation facilities, and yoga studios around the world, offering a gentle and inclusive approach to yoga practice for people of all ages and abilities.

Principles and Techniques of Chair Yoga

Chair yoga follows the same foundational principles as traditional yoga, with a focus on breath awareness, mindful movement, and relaxation. However, it adapts these principles to accommodate the seated position and use of a chair for support. Here are some key principles and techniques of chair yoga:

Breath Awareness: Like traditional yoga, chair yoga emphasizes the importance of conscious breathing. Practitioners are encouraged to focus on deep, diaphragmatic breathing, using the breath to anchor their awareness in the present moment and facilitate relaxation.

Mindful Movement: Chair yoga incorporates gentle movement sequences and modified yoga poses that are performed while seated on a chair or using a chair for support. These movements are designed to improve flexibility, mobility, and strength, while also promoting mindfulness and body awareness.

Adaptability: One of the defining features of chair yoga is its adaptability. Poses and sequences can be modified to suit individual needs, preferences, and physical limitations. Chairs can be used for support, balance, or stability, allowing practitioners to safely explore a wide range of movements and postures.

Safety and Comfort: Safety and comfort are paramount in chair yoga. Practitioners are encouraged to listen to their bodies, honor their limitations, and avoid pushing themselves beyond their comfort zone. Props such as blankets, blocks, and straps may be used to enhance comfort and support during practice.

Mind-Body Connection: Chair yoga fosters a deep connection between the mind and body, promoting greater self-awareness and self-acceptance. Through mindful movement and breath awareness, practitioners learn to cultivate a sense of presence, equanimity, and inner peace, both on and off the mat.

Relaxation and Meditation: Chair yoga often includes relaxation and meditation techniques to promote stress relief and mental wellbeing. Guided relaxation exercises, visualization, and mindfulness practices help practitioners release tension, quiet the mind, and cultivate a sense of calmness and relaxation.

Overall, chair yoga offers a gentle yet effective way to experience the benefits of yoga practice, regardless of age, fitness level, or physical ability. By honoring the body's needs and limitations, and embracing the principles of breath awareness, mindful movement, and relaxation, chair yoga empowers individuals to nurture their physical, mental, and emotional wellbeing in a safe and accessible manner.

Whether you're recovering from injury, managing a chronic condition, or simply looking for a gentle way to stay active and centered, chair yoga invites you to explore the transformative power of yoga from the comfort of your chair.

Adaptations to yoga practices for Men Over 50

As men age, their bodies undergo various changes that can impact their physical health, mobility, and overall wellbeing. While yoga offers numerous benefits for individuals of all ages, adapting yoga practice to meet the unique needs of men over 50 can enhance its effectiveness and accessibility. In this comprehensive guide, we will explore specific adaptations to yoga practice that cater to the needs of men in their prime years, empowering them to navigate physical changes with mindfulness and ease.

Before diving into adaptations to yoga practice, it's essential to understand the specific needs and challenges that men over 50 may face. Common issues include:

- Decreased flexibility and mobility due to changes in muscle elasticity, joint stiffness, and connective tissue tightness.

- Age-related muscle loss (sarcopenia) and decreased muscle strength, particularly in the core and lower body.

- Joint pain, arthritis, and other musculoskeletal conditions that may affect movement and comfort.

- Reduced balance and stability, increasing the risk of falls and injuries.

- Stress, anxiety, and other mental health concerns that may arise from life transitions, career changes, or retirement.

Adaptations to Yoga Practice

To address these specific needs and challenges, men over 50 can benefit from tailored adaptations to their yoga practice. Here are some key considerations and modifications:

Focus on Joint Health: Choose yoga poses and sequences that prioritize joint mobility and flexibility, such as gentle stretching movements and dynamic range-of-motion exercises. Avoid deep or intense stretches that may exacerbate joint pain or discomfort.

Build Strength Safely: Incorporate strength-building exercises into your yoga practice to counteract age-related muscle loss and maintain functional strength. Focus on core-strengthening poses, such as modified plank variations, chair squats, and leg lifts, using props or modifications as needed for support.

Mindful Movement: Practice yoga with mindful awareness, paying attention to sensations in the body and honoring your limitations. Avoid pushing yourself too hard or striving for perfection in poses. Instead, focus on moving with ease and grace, finding a balance between effort and relaxation.

Use Props for Support: Props such as blocks, straps, blankets, and chairs can provide additional support and stability during yoga practice. Use props as needed to modify poses, improve alignment, and reduce strain on joints and muscles.

Adapt Poses for Comfort: Modify yoga poses to suit your individual needs and physical limitations. For example, use a chair for seated poses or balance exercises, elevate the hips in seated forward bends to reduce strain on the lower back, or use a wall for support in standing poses.

Incorporate Breathwork and Relaxation: Integrate breath awareness, pranayama (breathing exercises), and relaxation techniques into your yoga practice to reduce stress, promote mental clarity, and enhance overall wellbeing. Practice deep, diaphragmatic breathing to calm the nervous system and cultivate a sense of inner peace.

Listen to Your Body: Above all, listen to your body and honor its signals during yoga practice. If a pose feels uncomfortable or causes pain, back off or modify as needed. Focus on finding a balance between effort and ease, allowing yourself to rest when necessary and respecting your body's limitations.

Chapter 2

Warm up Exercises

Neck Rolls

- Sit comfortably in a chair with your feet flat on the floor.
- Slowly drop your chin towards your chest and roll your head gently to the right, bringing your right ear towards your right shoulder.
- Hold for a few breaths, then roll your head back to center and repeat on the left side.
- Continue alternating sides for several repetitions, moving slowly and mindfully.

Shoulder Rolls

- Sit tall with your spine straight and shoulders relaxed.
- Inhale as you lift your shoulders up towards your ears, squeezing them tightly.
- Exhale as you roll your shoulders back and down in a smooth, circular motion.

- Repeat the shoulder rolls several times, alternating between forward and backward rotations.

Arm Circles

- Extend your arms out to the sides at shoulder height, palms facing down.
- Begin making small circles with your arms, moving them forward in a controlled motion.
- Gradually increase the size of the circles, allowing your shoulders to warm up and loosen.
- After a few repetitions, reverse the direction of the circles, moving your arms backward.

Wrist Rotations

- Extend your arms out in front of you, palms facing down.
- Slowly rotate your wrists in a circular motion, moving your hands clockwise.

- After a few rotations, switch to counterclockwise rotations.
- Continue the wrist rotations for several repetitions, focusing on loosening up the wrists and forearms.

Ankle Circles

- Extend your right leg out in front of you, keeping your foot flexed.
- Rotate your right ankle in a circular motion, moving clockwise.
- After a few rotations, switch to counterclockwise rotations.
- Repeat the ankle circles several times, then switch to the left leg and repeat the sequence.

Scan Code to download free bonus

Chapter 3

Position

Sit tall on the chair with feet hip-width apart, hands resting on thighs.

Steps

Lengthen the spine, relax your shoulders, and lift the crown of the head towards the ceiling.

Reps: Hold for 5-10 breaths.

Purpose

Improves posture and overall body awareness.

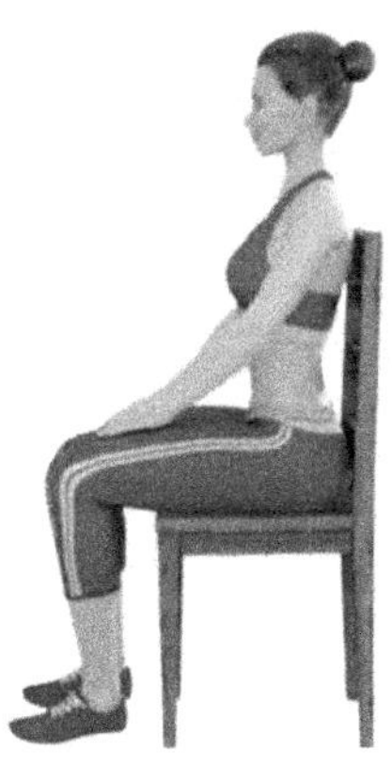

Position

Sit on the edge of the chair with feet flat on the floor.

Steps

Inhale to lengthen your spine, exhale to hinge at the hips and fold forward.

Reps: Hold for 5-8 breaths.

Purpose: Helpful for stretching the the spine, hamstrings, and shoulders.

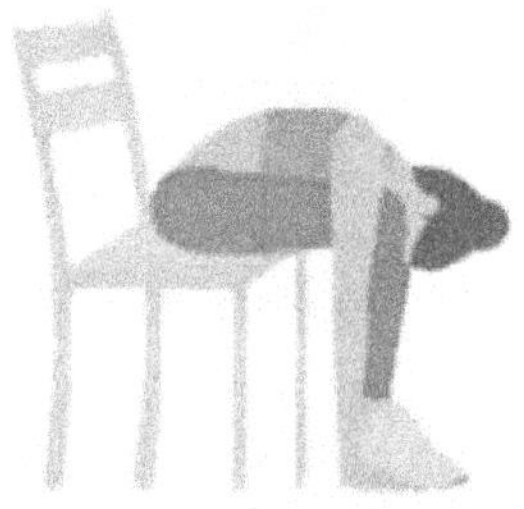

Position

Sit tall with your hands resting on your knees.

Steps

Inhale as you arch your back and lift your chest (cow pose), Exhale as you round your spine and tuck your chin towards your chest (cat pose). Flow between cat and cow poses with each breath for several repetitions.

Reps: Repeat 5-8 times.

Purpose: Improves spinal flexibility and mobility.

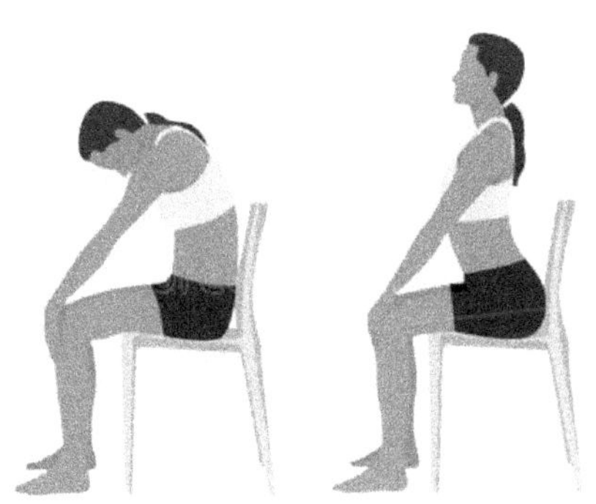

Position

Sit tall on the chair with feet flat on the floor.

Steps

Inhale as you lengthen your spine, exhale as you twist to one side, placing the opposite hand on the outside of the thigh.

Reps: Hold for 3-5 breaths on each side.

Purpose

Increases spinal mobility and aids digestion and promotes detoxification.

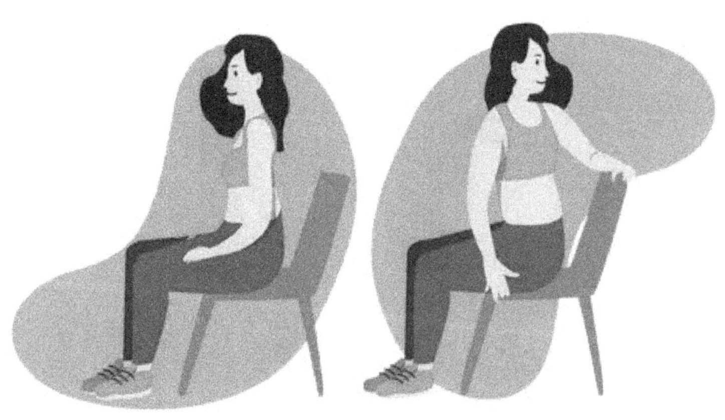

Position

Sit tall with your feet flat on the floor and your arms extended overhead.

Steps

Inhale to lengthen your spine, then exhale to lean to the right, reaching your left arm overhead. Hold the stretch for a few breaths, then repeat on the opposite side.

Reps:

Purpose

Helpful for stretching the side body, increasing flexibility, and relieving tension in the shoulders and waist.

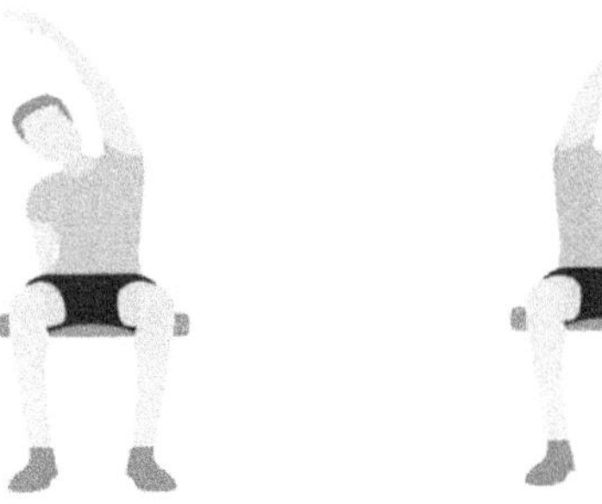

Position

Sit tall on the chair with feet flat on the floor.

Steps

Extend right leg back, keeping toes on the floor, and bend the left knee, stacking it over the ankle.

Reps: Hold for 3-5 breaths, then switch sides.

Purpose

Builds strength in the legs and opens the hips.

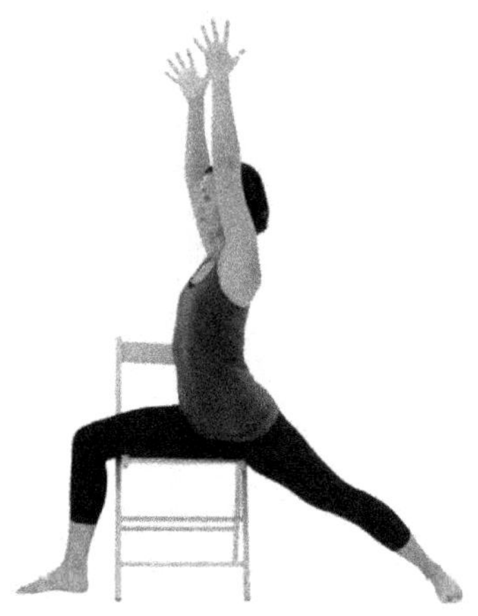

Position
Sit tall on the chair with feet flat on the floor.

Steps
Extend right leg back, keeping toes on the floor, and open the hips and chest to the right, extending arms out to the sides.

Reps: Hold for 3-5 breaths, then switch sides.

Purpose
Strengthens the legs and improves hip flexibility.

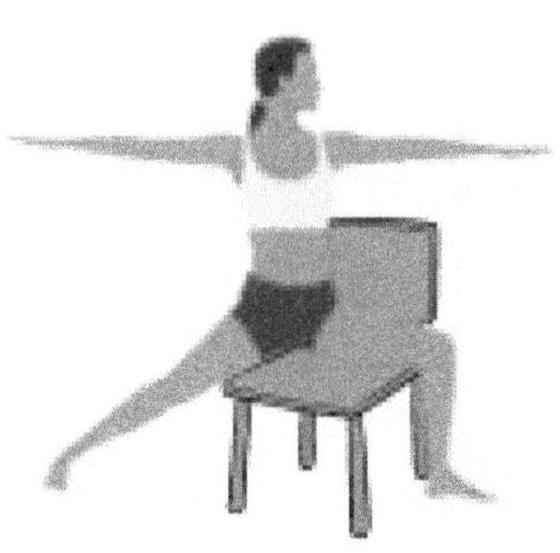

Position

Stand in front of the chair with feet flat on the floor.

Steps

Step right foot back, keeping toes on the floor, and press through the heel to lift the knee.

Reps: Hold for 3-5 breaths, then switch sides.

Purpose

Ideal for building strength in the legs and core, improving balance, and increasing hip flexibility.

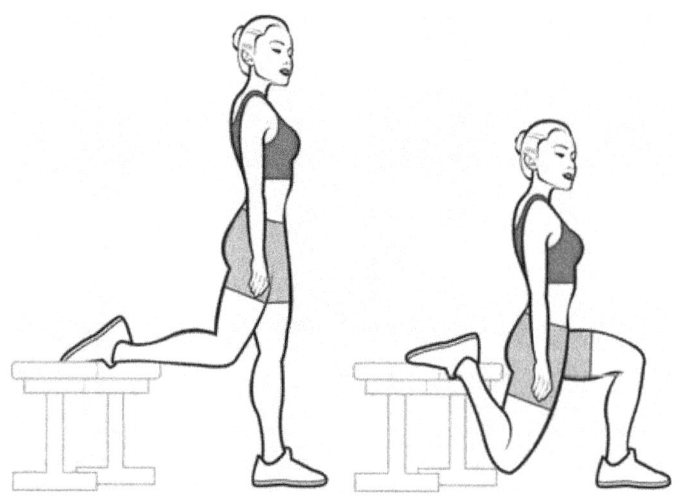

Position

Sit tall with your feet flat on the floor and your hands resting on your thighs.

Steps

Lift your right foot off the floor and place the sole of your right foot on your left inner thigh. Press your foot into your thigh and your thigh into your foot to create stability. Hold the pose for a few breaths, then repeat on the opposite side.

Reps: Hold for 5 breaths on each side

Purpose

Beneficial for improving balance and concentration, strengthening the legs.

Position

Sit tall with your feet flat on the floor.

Steps

Inhale as you sweep your arms out to the sides and overhead. Exhale as you cross your right arm under your left, wrapping your forearms around each other.

Bend forward at the hips, bringing your chest towards your thighs and your arms towards the floor. Hold the pose for a few breaths, then slowly return to an upright position and repeat with the opposite arm on top.

Reps: Hold for 5 breaths on each side

Purpose: Helpful for stretching the shoulders, upper back, and hamstrings, promoting relaxation and reducing tension.

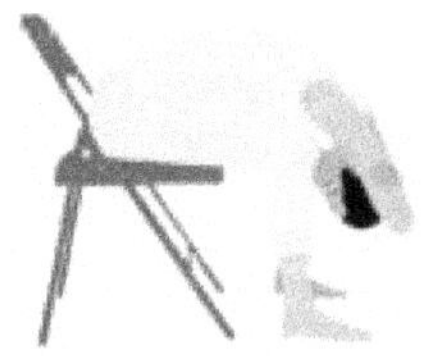

Position

Sit on a chair with your feet flat on the ground and knees bent at 90 degrees.

Steps

Start by placing your left hand on the left side of the chair's seat. Extend your right leg out to the side, keeping it straight. Reach your right arm up and over, stretching towards the left side. Hold the stretch for a few breaths. Repeat on the other side.

Reps: 3-5 repetitions on each side.
Purpose: Stretches and strengthens the side body, improves flexibility, and opens up the hips and shoulders.

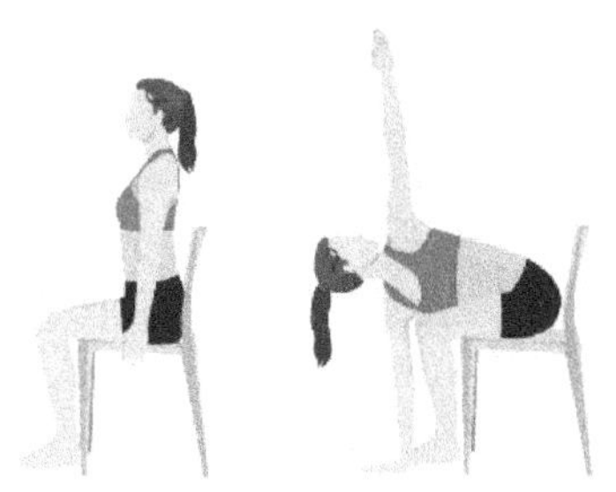

- Sit tall with your feet flat on the floor and your hands resting on your thighs.
- Inhale as you reach your arms out to the sides and lift them overhead.
- Exhale as you bend your elbows and bring your hands behind your head, clasping your hands together.
- Press your elbows back and lift your chest towards the ceiling, feeling a stretch across your chest and shoulders.
- Hold the pose for a few breaths, then release and repeat as desired.
- Ideal for relieving tension in the shoulders and upper back, improving posture, and reducing stress.

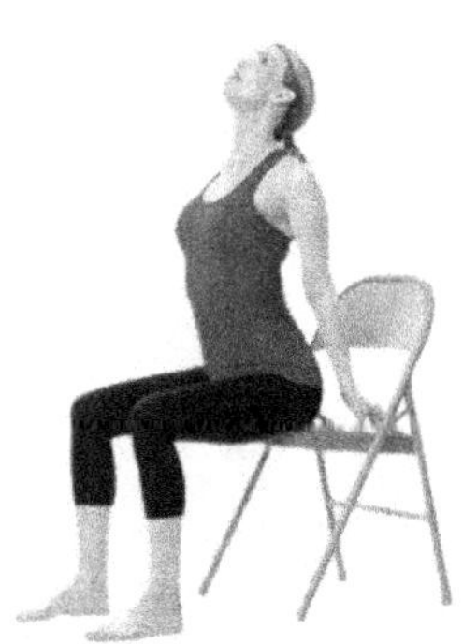

Position

Sit tall with your feet flat on the floor and your hands resting on your thighs.

Steps

Inhale as you lift your chest and gaze towards the ceiling, arching your back slightly. Press your palms into your thighs and engage your core. Hold the pose for a few breaths, then slowly release and return to an upright position.

Reps: Hold for 5 breaths

Purpose

Beneficial for strengthening the back muscles, improving spinal mobility, and relieving tension in the chest and shoulders.

Position

Sit towards the front edge of your chair with your feet flat on the floor.

Steps

Inhale as you lean back slightly, lifting your feet off the floor and extending your legs in front of you. Engage your core and lift your chest towards the ceiling, balancing on your sit bones.

Reps: Hold for 5 breaths and then slowly lower your feet back to the floor.

Purpose

Helpful for strengthening the core muscles, improving balance, and promoting abdominal strength and stability.

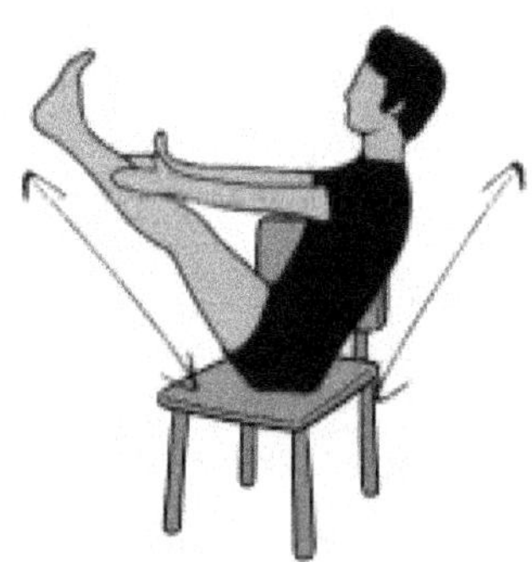

Position

Sit towards the front edge of your chair with your feet flat on the floor and your knees bent.

Steps

Inhale as you press down through your feet and lift your hips towards the ceiling. Engage your glutes and thighs to create stability.

Reps: Hold the pose for a 5 breaths, then slowly lower your hips back to the chair.

Purpose

Suitable for strengthening the glutes and hamstrings, improving lower back flexibility, and relieving tension in the spine.

Position

Sit towards the front edge of your chair with your feet flat on the floor and your knees bent.

Steps

Extend your right leg out in front of you, flexing your foot. Inhale as you tap your right toes to the floor, then exhale as you lift your leg back up.

Reps: Perform 10 reps on each leg

Purpose

Beneficial for strengthening the quadriceps, improving knee stability, and increasing lower body strength.

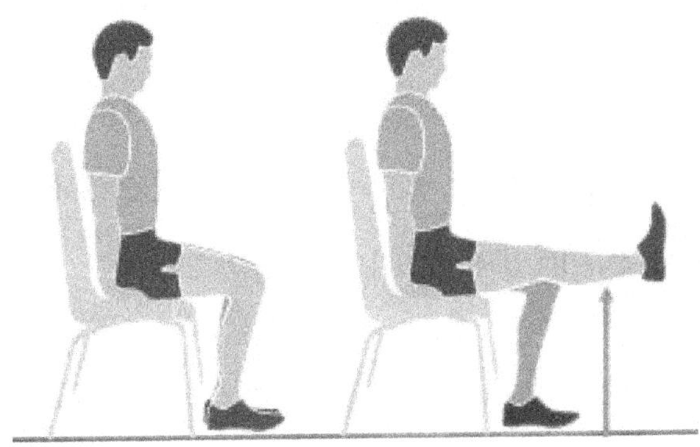

Position

Sit tall with your feet flat on the floor and your hands resting on your thighs.

Steps

Inhale as you lift your right knee towards your chest, clasping your hands around your knee. Exhale as you gently pull your knee closer to your chest, feeling a stretch in your hip and lower back.

Reps: Hold each leg for 5 breaths.

Purpose

Helpful for stretching the hips, lower back, and glutes, reducing tension and improving flexibility.

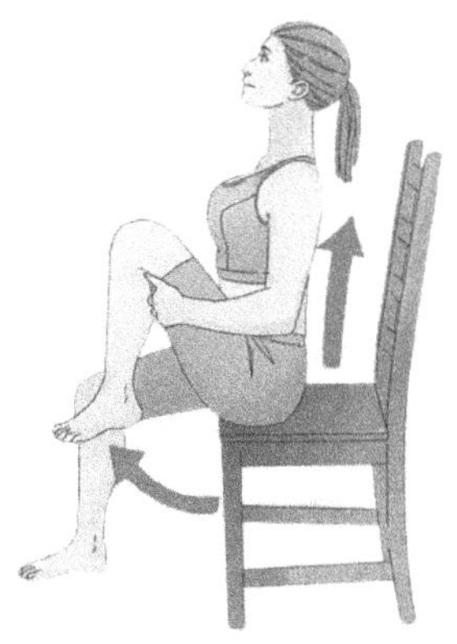

Position

Sit towards the front edge of your chair with your feet flat on the floor and your knees bent.

Steps

Extend your right leg out in front of you, keeping your foot flexed. Inhale as you lengthen your spine, then exhale as you hinge forward at the hips, reaching towards your right foot.

Reps: Hold the stretch for a few breaths, then return to an upright position and repeat on the opposite side.

Purpose

Suitable for stretching the hamstrings and calves, reducing tightness in the lower body, and improving flexibility.

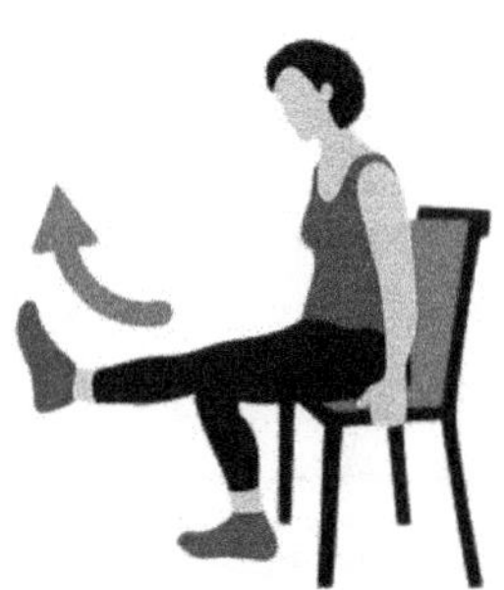

Position

Stand at the back of your chair with your feet flat on the floor.

Steps

Extend your right leg behind you and reach back with your right hand to grasp your right ankle. Gently pull your heel towards your glutes, feeling a stretch in the front of your thigh.

Reps: Hold the stretch for a 5 breaths, then release and repeat on the opposite side.

Purpose

Ideal for stretching the quadriceps, improving hip flexibility, and relieving tension in the thighs and knees.

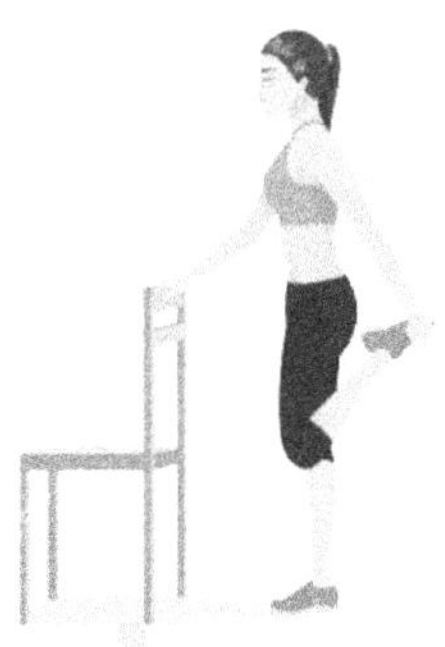

Position

Stand towards the back edge of your chair with your feet flat on the floor.

Steps

Extend your right leg out in front of you and flex your foot. Inhale as you press down through your right heel, lengthening your calf muscle.

Hold the stretch for a few breaths, then release and repeat on the opposite side.

Beneficial for stretching the calves, reducing tightness and discomfort, and improving ankle flexibility.

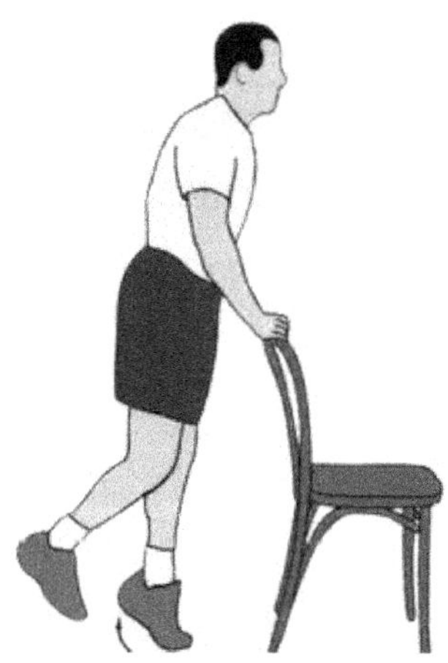

Position

Sit tall with your feet flat on the floor and your arms extended out to the sides.

Steps

Cross your right arm under your left, wrapping your forearms around each other. Press your palms together and lift your elbows towards the ceiling, feeling a stretch across your upper back and shoulders.

Reps: Hold pose for 5 breaths, then release and repeat with the opposite arm on top.

Purpose

Helpful for stretching the shoulders and upper back, improving posture, and reducing tension in the neck and shoulders.

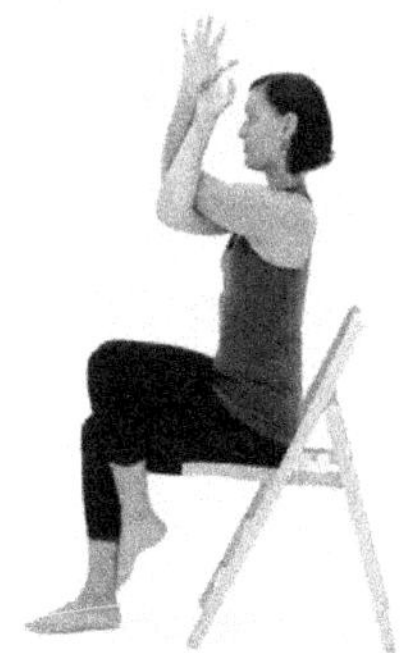

Position

Sit tall with your feet flat on the floor and your knees bent.

Steps

Inhale as you bring the soles of your feet together, allowing your knees to fall out to the sides. Hold onto your ankles or feet with your hands and lengthen your spine. Press your elbows into your thighs to deepen the stretch in your inner thighs and groin.

Reps: Hold the stretch for a few breaths, then release and repeat as desired.

Purpose

Suitable for stretching the inner thighs and groin, improving hip flexibility, and relieving tension in the hips and lower back.

Position

Sit tall with your feet flat on the floor and your hands resting on your thighs.

Steps

Inhale as you lift your shoulders up towards your ears, squeezing them tightly. Exhale as you roll your shoulders back and down in a smooth, circular motion.

Reps: Perform 10 repetitions, focusing on releasing tension in the shoulders and upper back.

Purpose

Ideal for releasing tension in the shoulders and upper back, improving posture, and reducing stress.

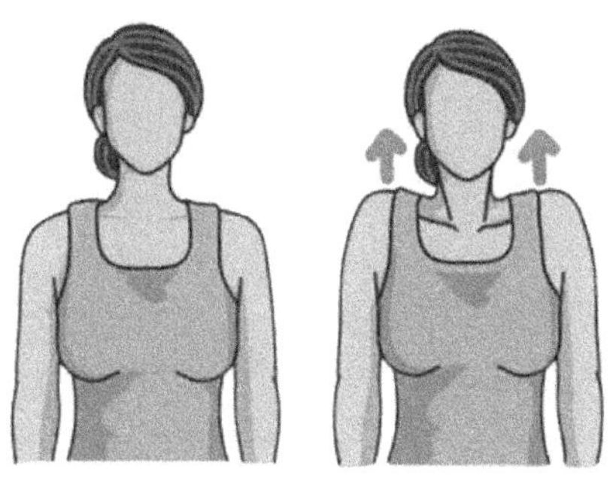

Position

Sit tall with your arms extended out in front of you and your palms facing down.

Steps

Begin making small circles with your wrists, moving clockwise. After a few rotations, switch to counterclockwise rotations.

Reps: perform 10 reps to loosening up the wrists and forearms.

Purpose

Beneficial for improving wrist mobility and flexibility, reducing stiffness, and relieving discomfort in the hands and forearms.

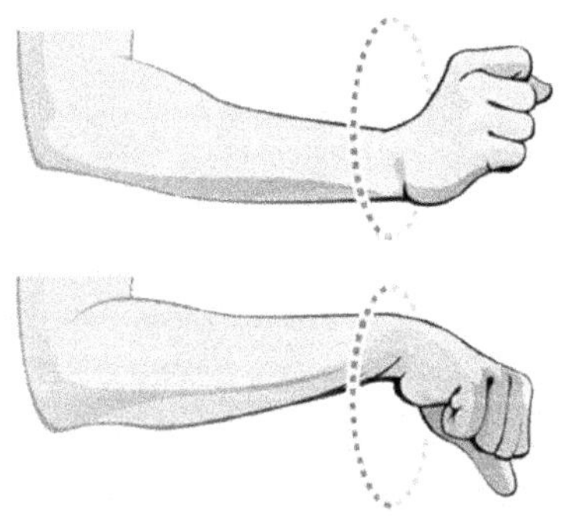

Position

Sit tall with your feet flat on the floor and your hands resting on your thighs.

Steps

Inhale as you lift your right leg off the floor, extending it out in front of you. Exhale as you lower your leg back down to the floor.

Reps: Repeat the leg lifts for 5 breaths, then switch legs and repeat on the opposite side.

Purpose

Helpful for strengthening the quadriceps and hip flexors, improving knee stability, and increasing lower body strength.

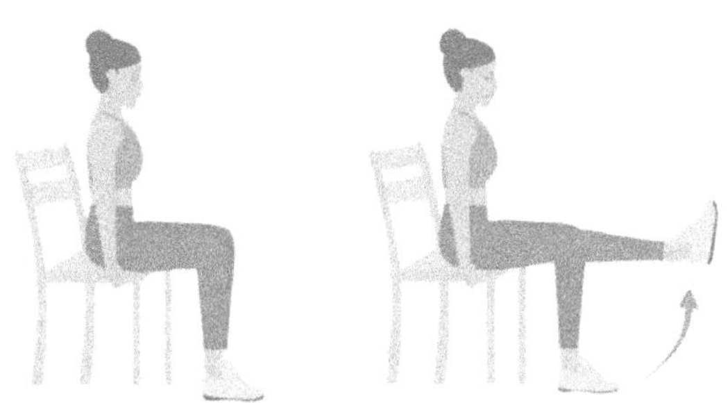

Position

Sit tall with your feet flat on the floor and your hands resting on your thighs.

Steps

Inhale as you extend your right leg out in front of you, keeping your foot flexed. Exhale as you bend your right knee and bring your foot back towards your body.

Reps: Repeat 10 times for each leg

Purpose

Suitable for strengthening the quadriceps and improving knee stability and mobility.

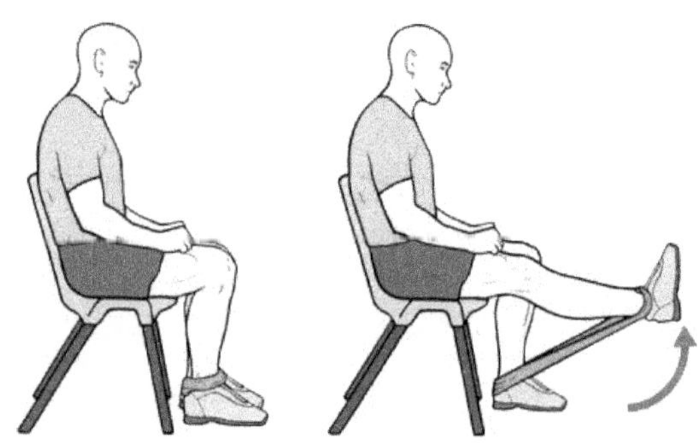

Position

Sit tall with your feet flat on the floor and your arms hanging down by your sides. Hold onto a pair of light weights or water bottles in each hand.

Steps

Inhale as you curl your hands towards your shoulders, bending at the elbows. Exhale as you lower your hands back down to the starting position.

Reps: repeat step 10 time to engage the biceps and maintaining good posture.

Purpose

Beneficial for strengthening the biceps, improving arm strength, and enhancing overall upper body strength and tone.

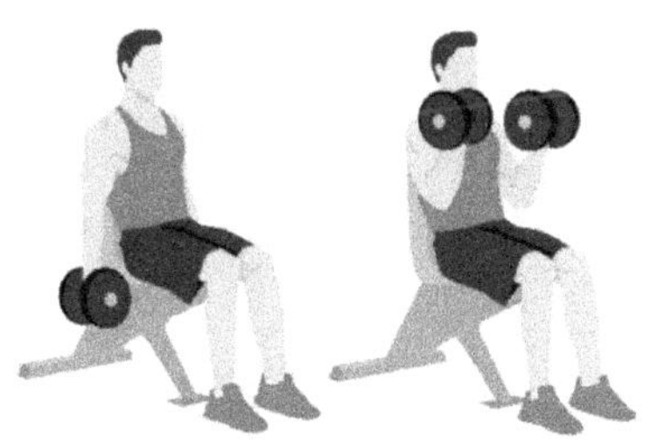

Position

Sit tall with your feet flat on the floor and your hands resting on the edge of your chair.

Steps

Slide your hips forward off the chair, keeping your hands planted firmly on the edge. Bend your elbows and lower your hips towards the floor, feeling a stretch in your triceps. Press down through your hands to lift your hips back up to the starting position.

Reps: Repeat the tricep dips 10 times.

Purpose

Suitable for strengthening the triceps and improving arm strength and tone, reducing the risk of injury.

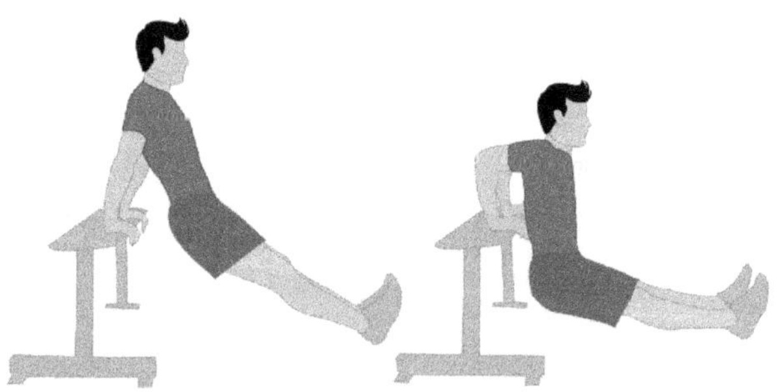

Position

Sit tall with your feet flat on the floor and your hands resting on your thighs.

Step

Close your eyes and take a few deep breaths

Purpose

Helpful for promoting relaxation, reducing stress and anxiety, and cultivating a sense of calm and wellbeing.

Position

Sit on a chair with your feet flat on the ground and spine tall.

Steps

Sit up straight with your feet flat on the ground. Lift your right arm straight up overhead. Bend your right elbow and reach your right hand down towards the center of your upper back. With your left hand, gently press down on your right elbow to deepen the stretch. Hold the stretch for 15-30 seconds.

Reps: 2-3 repetitions on each side.

Purpose

Stretches the shoulders, triceps, and upper back muscles, helps alleviate tension and improve flexibility in the shoulders, promotes better posture.

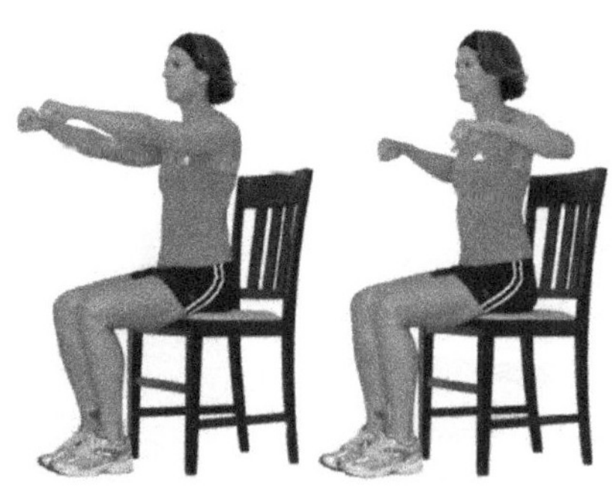

CONCLUSION

Yoga is not merely a physical practice, it is a comprehensive journey that include the mind, body, and spirit. Through the various poses, breathing techniques, and mindfulness practices outlined in this book, you have embarked on a transformative path towards self-discovery and well-being.

As you close this book, remember that yoga is not about perfection but about progress. Each time you step onto your mat, you have the opportunity to reconnect with yourself, cultivate awareness, and embrace the present moment with acceptance and compassion.

May the wisdom of yoga continue to guide you on your journey, both on and off the mat. Whether you are seeking strength, flexibility, inner peace, or simply a moment of stillness in a busy world, may you always find solace in the practice of yoga.

As you move forward, remember these words from B.K.S. Iyengar: "Yoga teaches us to cure what need not be endured and endure what cannot be cured." May your yoga practice empower you to navigate life's challenges with grace and resilience.

Thank you for allowing me to be a part of your yoga journey. May your path be filled with light, love, and endless possibilities.

Namaste.

[Maxwell Strong]